MW00902624

MEDICAL PRACTICE MANAGEMENT
Body of Knowledge Review

VOLUME 8

Professional Responsibility

David Peterson, MBA, FACMPE

Ken Mace, MA, CMPE

Managing Editor
Lawrence F. Wolper, MBA, FACMPE

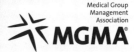

Medical Group
Management
Association

Medical Group Management Association
104 Inverness Terrace East
Englewood, CO 80112-5306
877.275.6462
Website: www.mgma.com

Medical Group Management Association (MGMA) publications are intended to provide current and accurate information and are designed to assist readers in becoming more familiar with the subject matter covered. Such publications are distributed with the understanding that MGMA does not render any legal, accounting, or other professional advice that may be construed as specifically applicable to an individual situation. No representations or warranties are made concerning the application of legal or other principles discussed by the authors to any specific factual situation, nor is any prediction made concerning how any particular judge, government official, or other person will interpret or apply such principles. Specific factual situations should be discussed with professional advisors.

Production Credits
Executive Editor: Andrea M. Rossiter, FACMPE
Managing Editor: Lawrence F. Wolper, MBA, FACMPE
Editorial Director: Marilee E. Aust
Production Editor: Marti A. Cox, MLIS
Substantive and Copy Editor: Sandra Rush, Rush Services
Proofreader: Scott Vickers, InstEdit
Page Design, Composition and Production: Boulder Bookworks
Cover Design: Ian Serff, Serff Creative Group, Inc.
MGMA Editorial Council Reviewer: Sabina Smith, CMPE

PUBLISHER'S CATALOGING IN PUBLICATION DATA

Peterson, David
    Professional responsibility / by David Peterson, Ken Mace ; managing editor Lawrence F. Wolper. – Englewood, CO : MGMA, 2006.
    64 p. ; cm. – (Medical Practice Management Body of Knowledge Review Series ; v. 8)
Includes index.
ISBN 1-56829-276-7
    1. Group practice administrators. 2. Ethics, Medical. 3. Ethics, Professional. [MeSH] 4. Medical personnel—Professional ethics. [LC] 5. Medical ethics. [LC] I. Mace, Ken. II. Wolper, Lawrence F. III. Medical Group Management Association. IV. American College of Medical Practice Executives. V. Series. VI. Series: Body of Knowledge Review Series.

R725.5.P48 2006
174.2—dc22   2005938862

Item 6359

ISBN: 1-56829-276-7   Library of Congress Control Number: 2005938862

Printed in the United States of America
10 9 8 7 6 5 4 3 2 1

Dedication

To Ingrid,
my personal and professional compass.
David Peterson

To my mentors and models,
whether they knew it or not…
Ken Mace

Contents

Series Overview

THE MEDICAL GROUP MANAGEMENT ASSOCIATION (MGMA) serves medical practices of all sizes, as well as management services organizations, integrated delivery systems, and ambulatory surgery centers to assist members with information, education, networking, and advocacy. Through the American College of Medical Practice Executives® (ACMPE®), MGMA's standard-setting and certification body, the organization provides board certification and Fellowship in medical practice management and supports those seeking to advance their careers.

- ■ **Core Learning Series: A professional development pathway for competency and excellence in medical practice management**

Medical practice management is one of the fastest-growing and most rewarding careers in health care administration. It is also one of the most demanding, requiring a breadth of skills and knowledge unique to the group practice environment. For these reasons, MGMA and ACMPE have created a comprehensive series of learning resources, customized to meet the specific professional development needs of medical practice managers: the *Medical Practice Management Core Learning Series*.

The Medical Practice Management Core Learning Series is a structured approach that enables practice administrators and staff to build the core knowledge and skills required for career success. Series resources include seminars, Web-based education programs, books, and online assessment tools. These resources provide a strong, expansive foundation for managing myriad job responsibilities and daily challenges.

■ Core Learning Series: Resources for understanding medical practice operations

To gain a firm footing in medical practice management, executives need a broad understanding of the knowledge and skills required to do the job. The Medical Practice Management Core Learning Series offers "Level 1" resources, which provide an introduction to the essentials of medical practice management. As part of the learning process, professionals can use these resources to assess their current level of knowledge across all competency areas, identify gaps in their education or experience, and select areas in which to focus further study. The *Medical Practice Management Body of Knowledge Review Series* is considered to be a Core Learning Series – Level 1 resource.

Level 1 resources meet the professional development needs of individuals who are new to or considering a career in the field of medical practice management, assuming practice management responsibilities, or considering ACMPE board certification in medical practice management.

Also offered are Core Learning Series – Level 2 resources, which provide exposure to more advanced concepts in specific competency areas and their application to day-to-day operation of the medical practice. These resources meet the needs of individuals who have more experience in the field, who seek specialized knowledge in a particular area of medical practice management, and/or who are completing preparations for the ACMPE board certification examinations.

■ Core Learning Series: Resources to become board certified

Board certification and Fellowship in ACMPE are well-earned badges of professional achievement. The designations Certified Medical Practice Executive (CMPE) and Fellow in ACMPE (FACMPE) indicate that the professional has attained significant levels of expertise across the full range of the medical practice administrator's responsibilities. The Medical Practice Management Core Learning Series is MGMA's recommended learning system for certification preparation. With attainment of the CMPE designation, practice executives will be well positioned to excel in their careers through ACMPE Fellowship.

Preface

DEALS GONE BAD, questionable business practices, and unorthodox decision making – every day the headlines alert us to these ethical lapses in judgment. The stories behind these headlines vary, but the theme is consistent. The behavior of an individual or group of individuals, or a corporate strategy of greed and short-sighted thinking, has adversely affected what were once formidable, respected companies. In the general corporate environment, Enron, WorldCom, Adelphi Communications, and Arthur Andersen come immediately to mind as identifiable companies that either did not survive scandal or have been mortally wounded by it. In the health care environment, HealthSouth is a prominent casualty, as are several pharmaceutical companies who have incurred heavy fines for failing to reveal the known harmful effects of medications or for illegal kickbacks.[1] Recently, a respected hospital in New York announced a civil settlement with the U.S. government involving a massive Medicaid billing fraud and agreed to a payment of almost one billion dollars over 12 years.[2]

In addition to the businesses themselves, casualties of such corporate mismanagement include the company leadership, employees, investors, and, in the case of health care, the patients and the general public at large. In the wake of such scandals, perhaps it is no coincidence that the former chairman of the Federal Reserve Board, Alan Greenspan, took the occasion of his 2005 commencement address at the Wharton School of Business to talk about the merits of hard work, frugality, and honesty.[3] More specifically, Chairman Greenspan stated that "material success is possible in this world, and far more satisfying, when it comes without exploiting others." Citing, among others, the aforementioned corporate scandals, Greenspan urged the Wharton graduates to "hold themselves to a high standard and not to cut corners." He went on to say that "trust and personal reputation" are important and that relying "on the word of those with whom we do business allows goods and services to be efficiently exchanged."[4]

Greenspan refers to it as trust. Some call it honesty. Others label it personal integrity. Some might even refer to it as character. Whatever "it" is called, these and other similar traits all might be found under the rubric of professional responsibility, and indeed, one of the domains within the *ACMPE Guide to the Body of Knowledge for Medical Practice Management* is Professional Responsibility.[5] In fact, one might argue that within the Technical/Professional Knowledge and Skills competency, the trait of professional responsibility is the common, unifying thread that connects the other seven domains found within the *Guide*: (1) Financial Management; (2) Human Resource Management; (3) Planning and Marketing; (4) Information Management; (5) Risk Management; (6) Governance and Organizational Dynamics; (7) Business and Clinical Operations; and (8) Professional Responsibility. Not unlike Adam Smith's theory of the "invisible hand"[6] – a force that guides individual behavior through society – professional responsibility might just be the invisible hand that touches upon and guides the medical practice executive through the other seven domains of medical practice leadership.

Moreover, one could argue that it is the absence of this guiding hand and the lack of personal responsibility that has caused the demise of so many companies and affected the lives of so many individuals. To state it more clearly, professional responsibility can be the factor that distinguishes success from failure and the factor that distinguishes a medical practice executive from other nonclinical health care employees.

Professional responsibility, however, is more than a collection of words. It is, in itself, its own "body of knowledge," an accumulation of learned behavior, habits, knowledge, and experiences that help a medical practice executive set policy and make decisions that affect the individual, the practice, and the community at large. In fact, evidence exists that such accumulations of experiences help individuals intuitively – even instinctively – arrive at the right conclusion, even given a limited set of data.[7]

In the pages that follow, professional responsibility and its various components are more clearly defined.

Learning Objectives

AFTER READING THIS VOLUME, the medical practice executive will be able to:

1. Articulate the definition of professionalism and recognize its value;

2. Learn a variety of tools that can be used for self-assessment;

3. Recognize the value of self-improvement, including how to advance one's career;

4. Manage the information overload, rise above detail, and recognize the larger picture;

5. Draw upon the knowledge of a cohort of other professionals in the field and recognize the value of their consultations;

6. Understand the power of a personal code of ethics;

7. Appreciate the value of mentoring to the mentee, the mentor, and the community at large;

8. Distinguish the difference between "doing the right thing" and "doing things right";

9. Define the role and importance of leadership in steering the practice's business decisions; and

10. Identify key professional responsibility issues from the following vignette.

The ABC Clinic

ABC CLINIC is a 100-physician multispecialty clinic based in a large urban area. The clinic consists of one large facility with two satellite offices, one located in the inner city and one in a rapidly growing outlying suburban area. The patient population has a wide age range – from children, adolescents, and adults, to senior citizens. The socioeconomic status of the patients is equally as varied, ranging from commercially well-insured to government-insured populations. The physician–administrator executive team comprises a physician, who serves as president and chief executive officer (CEO) of the practice, and an administrator, who serves as chief operating officer. Both executives are governed by a 13-physician board of directors and 5-physician executive committee. The group's fiscal year is the same as the calendar year.

The physicians are paid a base salary plus an incentive. Incentives based on the physician's productivity are paid quarterly, and incentives based on the group's overall profitability are paid on the last day of each month. All payments to partners and staff physicians are governed by a written compensation plan adopted by the board of directors several years ago.

Recently, several requests have come to the CEO from physician partners regarding incentive payments. Partner One is going through a lengthy divorce and has requested that her incentive payments be deferred and that she receive only her base salary for the next year. Partner Two has asked that the check for his incentive payment, normally received on December 31, be paid on January 1 because he already has several personal taxable events in the current tax year. Partner Three has wondered if his incentive payments will increase if he makes more referrals to the group's affiliated hospital, orders more lab tests, or charges a higher fee to his especially well-heeled patients who are willing to pay a premium for his services. Partner Three's request to charge higher fees to some of his patients is in contrast to another partner's request that he be allowed to charge a lower fee to his patients who do not have insurance. Partner Three has also announced that he will no longer accept referrals from the practice's inner city satellite due to the lower payer mix of that patient panel, arguing that seeing patients from that practice hurts his income. These two partners' requests represent deviations from the group's adopted usual and customary fees.

In addition to these incentive payment requests, the CEO has received a request from the group's education director for practice funds to support a three-day retreat at his mountain lodge. The event would be catered, and the director and key support staff would be flown by private jet, at the practice's expense. The education director has also made arrangements with a pharmaceutical representative to have the pharmaceutical company pick up half the cost of the private jet.

Lastly, one of the practice's senior nurses, a long-time and valuable employee, burst into the CEO's office yesterday in tears, claiming that the newest partner's brusque, demanding, and offensive verbal style was creating an environment in which it was impossible to work. She stated that if the new partner's style doesn't change, she will either demand to be reassigned or will have to leave the practice after some 20 years of employment.

The CEO wants to take these questions to the executive committee, but has asked the administrator for an opinion and recommendation regarding each of the requests.

How the administrator responds may depend significantly on the knowledge of and sensitivity to the principles of professional responsibility outlined in the following pages. See the "Vignette Redux" later in this volume for a review of the key considerations in this scenario.

Professional Responsibility and the General Competencies

ACMPE HAS IDENTIFIED five general competencies that are expected of the medical practice executive: Professionalism, Leadership, Communication Skills, Organizational and Analytical Skills, and Technical/Professional Knowledge and Skills.[8] Without a doubt, professional responsibility is an essential component of each of these general competencies.

Professional responsibility defines, by its nature, professionalism. Tasks such as assessing oneself, balancing workflow, doing the "right thing," and giving back to the profession are embodied in the trait of professional responsibility.

Professional responsibility empowers leadership, providing credibility and a knowledge base that inspires the group practice. Awareness of organizational dynamics governance, the development of cutting-edge technologies, and knowledge of new business practices and trends enhance leadership, decision making, and authority.

Professional responsibility magnifies communication skills. The professionally active individual develops active listening skills, the know-how to knowledgeably present ideas, and the ability to identify the tools to sell ideas – essential components for a successful medical practice executive.

Professional responsibility sharpens organizational and analytical skills by providing a solid foundation and framework for practice management, analysis, and development.

Finally, as this volume shows, professional responsibility is the hand that guides the medical practice executive through the eight domains identified under the competency of Technical/Professional Knowledge and Skills.

Current Professional Responsibility Issues

IN THE HEALTH CARE FIELD, abbreviations, shorthand references, and acronyms are ubiquitous. HIPAA (Health Insurance Portability and Accountability Act of 1996), *qui tam*, Stark, safe harbors, Sarbanes-Oxley, and intermediate sanctions are a few examples of efforts by regulatory agencies to bring, among other things, accountability, transparency, and some semblance of fairness or equality to business and health care organizations. Such efforts are not only endless, they can be threatening as well because, if ignored, the organization and its leadership are vulnerable to sanctions, fines, and/or imprisonment.

Sarbanes-Oxley, for example, has been labeled the "single most important piece of legislation affecting corporate governance, financial disclosure and the practice of public accounting since the U.S. securities laws of the early 1930s."[9] Major provisions of the act include criminal and civil penalties for securities violations, auditor independence, and increased disclosure requirements.[10] The Stark and Stark II laws, named after the original sponsor of the legislation, Congressman Pete Stark (D-CA), govern physician self-referrals for Medicare and Medicaid patients. Stark covers 11 different categories for which physicians might questionably self-refer, ranging from clinical laboratory services to radiology, inpatient, and outpatient services.[11,12] The not-so-obvious problem Stark addresses is the opportunity for physicians to enrich themselves by ordering medical or ancillary services from corporate entities in which they have a financial interest.

HealthSouth agreed to pay a civil settlement of $100 million with the Securities and Exchange Commission to settle fraud allegations, in addition to previous settlements of $325 million to the Department of Justice and $80 million to bondholders. Richard Scrushy, HealthSouth CEO, was acquitted of charges filed against him under Sarbanes-Oxley.[13]

The headlines are full of these types of stories, which are indicative of the legislative and ethical minefield through which the medical practice executive needs to navigate. However, the domain of professional responsibility extends far beyond an awareness and knowledge of legislative initiatives. A broad knowledge base and an awareness of issues and current events are necessary for the medical practice executive. For example, medical practices and health care organizations are vulnerable to *qui tam* actions, which are actions brought by interested third parties (whistle-blowers) on behalf of someone else, usually the federal government.[14] Medical practice leadership might be held liable under the doctrine of *respondeat superior*, a doctrine of law that holds employers liable for their employee's actions.[15]

Under the Federal Anti-Kickback Statute and the Stark laws, safe harbors exist to protect the physician and the practice. Safe harbors can shield the group from regulatory or legal action, and failure to recognize and take advantage of a safe harbor provision places the physician and the practice at risk.[16]

Awareness of these and other components in the professional responsibility domain is essential for the medical practice executive. Recognizing hostile vs. family-friendly work environments, balancing work and family commitments, pursuing continuing education, developing and maximizing an interpersonal skill set, effectively using professional networks, managing time, and capitalizing on other professional resources and techniques are all elements of the domain that are critical to the health care leader's success. A broad knowledge of the field protects not only the practice, but the medical practice executive as well. In human resources, for example, well-intentioned but too generous employee salaries and benefits might lead to Intermediate Sanctions for the leadership of a nonprofit, 501(c)3 corporation.[17] In fact, the law explicitly mandates that the penalties for Intermediate Sanctions be personally borne by the leadership and that they cannot be compensated by the practice.[18]

That same broad knowledge set is necessary to recognize gaps that require the medical practice executive to seek outside expert assistance when necessary. The labyrinth of laws, regulations, and rules are sometimes too complex, and the penalties for violating them are often too severe for the informed amateur to try and understand, implement, or work around. It is a common tenet that "ignorance of the law is no defense"[19]; thus, recognizing complexity when complexity exists and seeking appropriate outside expertise are trademarks of the successful professional medical practice executive.

In short, the domain of Professional Responsibility is broad and far-reaching. Just as the medical practice executive can personally touch many lives – be they patients, employees, investors, or the community at large – the scope of knowledge and skill sets demanded by these same publics is equally as extensive.

Knowledge Needs

■ Professional Responsibility Knowledge Overview

As previously noted, it is relatively easy in both the business world and in health care to observe occasions in which a lack of professional responsibility has led to scandals, business failures, and even criminal behavior. Part of exercising professional responsibility is the necessity to answer the question, "What is professional responsibility?" Deconstructing this phrase leads one to better understand just how important professional responsibility is among the domains of the medical practice executive.

Responsibility simply means "to be responsible," which is defined in the *Oxford English Dictionary* as to be:

1. Legally or morally obligated to take care of something or to carry out a duty, liable to be blamed for loss or failure, etc.;

2. Having to account for one's actions, *you will be responsible to the president himself*;

3. Capable of rational conduct;

4. Trustworthy, *a responsible person*;

5. Involving important duties, *a responsible position*; or

6. Being the cause of something, *the plague was responsible for many deaths*.[20]

Clearly, a medical practice executive is in a responsible position and is accountable to many. But, responsibility alone does not also imply professionalism, and the definition of professionalism is much murkier than that of responsibility.

The definition of a profession or professionalism is as varied as the number of professions or would-be professions. A recent white paper on professionalism by MGMA and ACMPE quoted no less than 10 different definitions of professionalism.[21] Almost every defined occupational category that requires specific education has an association that carries its own group's definitions. Although the many definitions differ, they all have a set of common core values.

For example, the Florida Bar Association's Center for Professionalism carries on its Website the following statement:

Professionalism includes:

1. A *commitment* to serve others;

2. Being *dedicated* to proper use of one's knowledge to promote a *fair and just* result;

3. Endeavoring always to *enhance one's knowledge and skills*;

4. Ensuring that concern for the desired result does not subvert *fairness, honesty, respect, and courtesy* for others with whom one comes into contact, be they fellow professionals, clients, opponents, or public officials, including members of the judiciary or public;

5. *Contributing* one's skill, knowledge, and influence as a lawyer to further the profession's commitment to serving others and to *promoting the public good*, including efforts to provide all persons, regardless of their means or popularity of their causes, with access to the law and the judicial system;

6. *Educating* the public about the capabilities and limits of the profession, specifically what it can achieve and the appropriate methods of obtaining those results; and

7. *Accepting responsibility* for one's own professional conduct as well as that of others in the profession, including inculcat-

ing a desire to uphold professional standards and fostering peer regulation to ensure each member is competent and public spirited.[22]

The Accreditation Council for Graduate Medical Education (ACGME) defines professionalism as one of the core competencies to be taught in the training of physicians, and in its definition states:

> Residents must demonstrate a commitment to carrying out professional responsibilities, adherence to ethical principles, and sensitivity to a diverse patient population. Residents are expected to demonstrate respect, compassion and integrity; a responsiveness to the needs of patients and society that supersedes self-interest; accountability to patients, society and the profession; and a commitment to excellence and ongoing professional development. Residents are expected to demonstrate a commitment to ethical principles pertaining to provision or withholding of clinical care, confidentiality of patient information, informed consent, and business practices. Residents are expected to demonstrate sensitivity and responsiveness to patient's culture, age, gender and disabilities.[23]

The Australian Council of Professions puts forth this definition:

> A profession is a disciplined group of individuals who adhere to ethical standards and uphold themselves to, and are accepted by the public as possessing special knowledge and skills in a widely recognized body of learning derived from research, education and training at a high level, and who are prepared to exercise this knowledge and these skills in the interest of others. It is inherent in the definition of a profession that a code of ethics governs the activities of each profession. Such codes require behavior and practice beyond the personal moral obligations of an individual. These codes are enforced by the profession and are acknowledged and accepted by the community.[24]

Finally, the *Oxford English Dictionary* definition of a profession is:

> An occupation whose core element is work based upon the mastery of a complex body of knowledge and skill. It is a vocation in which knowledge of some department of science or learning or the practice of an art founded upon it is used in the service of others. Its members profess a commitment to competence, integrity and morality, altruism and the promotion of public good within their domain. These commitments form a basis of a social contract between a profession and a society, which in return grants the profession the right to autonomy in practice and the privilege of self-regulation. Professions and their members are accountable to those served and to society.[25]

Whether examining the definitions of professionalism from attorneys, physicians, teachers, or even the Reflexology Association of America, common themes emerge. Clearly, to be a professional requires:

- A mastery of a certain body of knowledge;
- Acceptance of a code of ethics, a willingness to put others' interests ahead of one's own;
- Commitment to continuing education; and
- In many cases, commitment to furthering one's field or body of knowledge.

The question that then arises involves whether medical practice management is a profession or only an occupation. In many ways medical practice management does rise to the level of a profession, but only when the practitioner accepts the challenge of professional responsibility. A medical practice manager who has neither studied the *ACMPE Guide to the Body of Knowledge for Medical Practice Management* nor adopted a code of ethics would not rise to the same level as a professional medical practice executive who has done those things. Is the medical practice executive seen as a professional by the community? In some cases, yes, but not universally – not in those cases where no accountability to the greater society has been accepted.

Thus, the conclusion is that by accepting professional responsibility, a medical practice executive can elevate himself or herself to a level of professionalism equal to that of the physician partners in the group practice, but attainment of that level of trust and respect must be a conscious choice or decision to accept the higher-level responsibilities of the professional.

■ Self-Assessment and Improvement

All definitions of professionalism include the need for ongoing education, but to match such education with needs, the medical practice executive must first undergo a self-assessment. Self-assessment is an ongoing process, not a simple one-time exercise. To perform effectively in any position, one learns to anticipate future needs and to then reflect upon how those needs match one's own current skill set. No one knows everything, and everyone benefits from ongoing education, but education is best leveraged when it is targeted at needs. To define needs, one has to recognize one's own strengths and weaknesses through the process of self-assessment. By inventorying one's skills against the entire ACMPE *Guide*, one can seek out those educational experiences that complement rather than reinforce one's existing skill set. The medical practice management body of knowledge is so broad and the subject so complex that there are always opportunities to learn more about a topic, especially when the pace of change is as high as it is in health care.

This high pace of change in health care requires continual, ongoing professional development for the medical practice executive. Not only are new skills needed on an ongoing basis, but whole new knowledge sets are continually being developed, refined, and updated. Just 10 years ago, who had ever heard of the now-common HIPAA legislation, and prior to 2004, who really believed there would be a Medicare drug benefit on the horizon? To effectively administer medical practices, the medical practice executive is constantly challenged to learn new things now, not someday. As noted in James D. Murphy's book, *Business Is Combat*, "if you're not computer literate now, get literate tonight"[26] because tomorrow you'll need to hit the ground running on that new information technology (IT) project.

Along with the need to continually acquire new knowledge, the medical practice executive needs to consider the advancement and certification process of ACMPE. By committing to the board certification advancement process, a medical practice executive is committing to mastering the *ACMPE Guide to the Body of Knowledge for Medical Practice Management*, and by accepting its Professional Responsibility domain, the executive is also committing to the goal of lifelong learning and continuing professional development. By progressing to Fellowship status in ACMPE, the medical practice executive is further committing to one of the highest levels of professionalism, contributing to the body of knowledge by developing three case studies or a professional paper.

Medical practice takes place in a certification-dominated world. MDs, DOs, PhDs, NPs, and PAs, to name a few, are all certified within their disciplines as competent to practice, and most specialties require meeting ongoing continuing-education requirements to maintain certification status. ACMPE's process is similar to that of the other disciplines or professions involved in health care, and by achieving board certification and then Fellowship status in ACMPE, the medical practice executive is demonstrating a commitment to professionalism comparable to that of those with whom he or she is working. Lastly, through the ACMPE advancement process, the executive can lay out and execute a long-range plan of personal achievement and professional growth by accumulating continuing education credits, making presentations, and contributing to the medical practice management body of knowledge.

■ Information Overload Management

Another key knowledge area of professional responsibility is managing the information overload and stress that occur in the health care field and life in general. The effective medical practice executive rises above the continual stream of new information and daily stressors to understand the context and the trends that are shaping the day-to-day decisions being made. "Thinking ahead," or what economist Thomas Sowell calls the "second stage" of thinking and understanding – how decisions lead from one to another and, even more critically, how different decisions lead to different sets of opportunities or risks in the future – is how the medical practice executive effectively leads the organization.[27] Continually asking the strategic question "What business is the group in?" is one way the thoughtful and effective executive provides leadership value to the group. This strategy includes evaluating alternative courses of action for both their long-term fit with the organization and with the strategic direction in which the organization is moving, as opposed to chasing every business opportunity that presents itself.[28] According to one consultant, "Great leaders avoid the bane of multi-taskers by resisting the addictive tendency to run around putting out brush fires rather than staying focused on what's important. They avoid the caffeinated tyranny of the urgent to follow through and complete what is truly significant."[29]

Information Networking and Mentoring

Along with the ability to think long-term, the effective executive also develops a cohort of colleagues, mentors, and coaches both in and out of the field and utilizes that network to reality-test his or her perceptions, understandings, and ideas. It is not uncommon for the effective executive to consult with other professionals or businesspeople about areas in which the expertise of the consultant is deeper than that of the more broadly trained practice executive. Consulting with attorneys, insurers, underwriters, financial professionals, architects, or even interior designers is a regular experience in the practice executive's business day. It is not uncommon for executives to discuss with others in the field different ways to approach problems. Every practice need not reinvent the wheel when a simple call to, or a cup of coffee with, a colleague might provide a mini-primer on how to approach a particular issue. Even though every practice is different, similar approaches work for multiple practices because the business environments in which practices operate are highly regulated and systematic.

Related to consulting with peers or experts is the concept of mentoring others. Professional executives recognize the value to the community, to themselves, and to junior colleagues of passing along accumulated wisdom, skills, tactics, and approaches. Along with avoiding the reinvention of the wheel, senior executives know that by passing along knowledge to subordinates and colleagues alike, one creates more effective organizations in the long run, a more well-trained community, and a more prepared group of eventual successors. Junior executives often identify one or more senior executives from whom to gain wisdom about the practice environment, career planning, specific management techniques, and even managing the work-life balance. Although the mentor/mentee relationship can sometimes turn destructive or become an exercise in ego, the community realizes value by having seniors train juniors, much as trades were traditionally passed from fathers to sons for hundreds of years before the modern economy.

■ Ethics and Leadership

One essential component of mentoring is teaching the value of having an ethical approach to one's responsibilities as a medical practice executive. The great majority of the decisions a practice executive makes involves not only technical, but moral and ethical choices as well. In fact, even the choices about which decisions to make have a moral or ethical component.

Ethical choices usually involve the various duties a practice executive must exercise in the course of the day. For instance, an executive has a duty to the partners to see that the practice is run economically and in conformance with the law. There is a duty to the employees that they be provided a safe work environment. There is a duty to the patients that their interests will be paramount in decisions on their care, to include confidentiality, clinical efficacy, and billing integrity, to name a few. Thus, having a strong set of ethical values actually makes some decisions and choices easier because it excludes certain decision outcomes that conflict with duty.

In the vignette at the beginning of this volume, the administrator is faced with several ethical issues that will guide his or her recommendations. There are legal conflicts in the partners' bonus and tax arrangement requests, there are conflicts of interest inherent in the proposed mountain retreat, and there is a duty to provide the veteran nurse with a safe work environment. In many ways following a strong ethical code is referred to as "doing the right thing vs. doing things right." A technically sound implementation of an unethical decision can lead to negative consequences just as rapidly as a wrong decision. Just as the executive must continually ask strategic questions, he or she must also ask of each decision, "What are the ethical impacts of this decision upon our partners, our employees, our patients, and our community?"

For example, compensation plans and fee schedules can be seen as numbers-driven mathematical exercises without ethical aspects. A poorly designed compensation plan could result in unfair treatment of partners or co-workers, in turn creating acrimony and disincentives, or in the worst case, providing incentives to leave the practice. Similarly, a poorly considered fee schedule could have the effect of pricing certain partners out of the market, or making certain services so expensive that they are never provided, regardless of their clinical efficacy.

Poorly designed fee schedules can also have the effect of "starving the practice" when fees are set well below what third-party payers are willing to pay. This results in a negative effect on the practice and, ultimately, the partners' incomes. Poorly designed fee schedules can also have the effect of placing needed services out of the financial reach of patients. Even in these more mundane fiscal policy-setting practices, therefore, "doing the right thing" becomes important. The testing and modeling of such schemes can reveal unintended consequences that could lead to potential conflict. Testing and modeling are among the most important tools for the professional medical practice executive. The essence of ethics and leadership is knowing the probable effects of decisions before these decisions are implemented.

In his 1989 film *Do the Right Thing*, director Spike Lee continuously employed the shout "Wake Up, Wake Up!" to spur individuals to continuously explore the ethical impacts of their actions.[30] In that critically acclaimed film, various characters go through the day without regard to the incremental impacts of their actions upon others, ultimately leading to disaster. Lee's film makes the point that every action one takes carries with it the responsibility for the outcome and that every action has an ethical dimension that needs to be considered. Throughout the day in the medical practice management field, the practice executive makes decisions, all of which carry ethical implications. Being guided by a strong set of ethical principles not only makes many decisions easier (because unethical options are ruled out), but makes them better because they lead to doing the right thing. It is difficult to imagine what two leaders of New York City's Health and Hospitals Corporation were thinking in 2005 when they admitted to accepting large personal loans from vendors as well as failing to transmit results of abnormal lab tests to patients. Both, of course, lost their jobs.[31]

The payoff from "doing the right thing" is one example of how an executive demonstrates leadership within the medical practice. Medical practice executives are not mere managers who function as hired help, doing whatever the partners ask. Effective executives are participants and leaders in the practice's decision-making processes. Physicians and providers often are not versed in the skills contained within the ACMPE *Guide*, and they expect the executive to bring that knowledge to the table. By providing this expertise and assisting in analysis and decision making, the skilled executive improves the practice, and by demonstrating that leadership the executive is recognized by the partners, the staff, and the community as a leader.

Overview of Professional Responsibility Tasks

MEDICAL PRACTICE EXECUTIVES must develop and use their knowledge and skills to ensure that the following tasks related to professional responsibility are carried out:

■ TASK 1: **Advance professional knowledge and leadership skills**

This task discusses the importance of assessing educational needs and why it is necessary to plan career advancement, with an emphasis on how to advance the medical practice management profession.

■ TASK 2: **Balance professional and personal pursuits**

To effectively maintain psychological and physical well-being, this task addresses the body-mind connection and why health and fitness are integral parts of every successful professional's routine.

■ TASK 3: Promote ethical standards for individual and organizational behavior and decision making

This task recognizes the need to develop individual and organizational integrity, implement ethical behaviors and goals into the practice's organizational culture, and set standards for ethical behavior, professionalism, and responsibility to the community. It also identifies the associated risks when ethics are ignored or abused.

■ TASK 4: Conduct self-assessments

This task shows how to identify the programs and resources necessary for setting and meeting competency requirements, including professional knowledge and skill assessments and personality classification models. The various assessment techniques are covered, as well as the importance of group and personal dynamics.

■ TASK 5: Engage in professional networking

This task presents the components and factors necessary to develop a system to classify jobs. This system will allow a better understanding of the dynamics necessary to have a workforce that meets marketplace demands.

■ TASK 6: Advance the profession by contributing to the body of knowledge

Which organizations in today's marketplace are best suited to assist a person with his or her next career step? Knowledge of existing professional organizations and networks as well as opportunities for coaching and mentoring is extremely important. This task addresses how to advance the profession through these avenues.

■ TASK 7: **Develop effective interpersonal skills**

The application of knowledge and skills to medical practice management as well as the ability to share knowledge and information with the profession are covered by this task. Perspectives on ambulatory medicine, practice management, community health care organizations, and health care issues are also included here.

TASK 1 **Advance Professional Knowledge and Leadership Skills**

■ Changing Information Requirements

One of the many facets that make medical practice management both challenging and rewarding is the incredible rate of change in the medico-economics field. New drugs and therapies, new surgical procedures, and new regulatory reforms are announced every day. All of the new drugs and procedures need to be factored into the microeconomic side of the health care equation, and the regulatory changes affect practices at all levels, from how one recruits new physician partners down to how the medical record clerk angles his or her computer screen. From the practice executive's perspective, these changes present both a challenge and an opportunity. There is no central oversight of medical practice, no universal implementers of new policies or procedures. Accordingly, it is up to the practice executive to keep abreast of all these changes, so that he or she can incorporate change into the practices in ways that are economical, affordable, and compliant with any new laws and regulations.

■ Change Management through Continuing Education

Medical practice executives not only need to implement a specific solution to each new change, but, equally important, they need to establish context for change. Often, staff – and even partners – are so absorbed in their own functions that they are not aware of larger trends in the health care or business environment. The executive must continue to monitor trends and stay up to date in order to establish context when asking staff or partners to make changes. Knowing there is a Medicare prescription drug benefit, and knowing both how the benefit works and how it is paid for, can help the executive communicate with partners and staff regarding prescribing patterns. Understanding the Internal Revenue Service (IRS) Intermediate Sanctions can help an executive in the nonprofit sector clarify why additional documentation and scrutiny of business-related expenses are necessary. Understanding the status of class-action lawsuits against hospitals regarding billing practices for the uninsured helps the executive explain why inquiries are being made regarding the group's practices around billing the uninsured.

Executives can keep up with information and change in many ways. The primary methods involve memberships and continuing education. Memberships in such groups as MGMA, ACMPE, and HFMA (Healthcare Financial Management Association) provide material such as monthly journals and electronic discussion groups, many tailored to specific needs. In addition, MGMA offers its members access to an online Knowledge Center, a Web portal providing access to literature databases, an article archive, and other information, as well as information products on specific topics, which can be ordered as needed. Every specialty publishes a variety of journals that offer articles and advice regarding practice management issues. In addition, a plethora of nonspecialty-specific journals are aimed at assisting the medical practice with its business, on issues ranging from coding alerts to medical economics. In many cases, monitoring the general press and business press (the daily newspaper, the *Wall Street Journal*, *Business Week*, and *Newsweek*, to name a few) can give an executive tips on upcoming knowledge needs, issues, and trends. Most professional organizations also sponsor numerous continuing-education events at which executives can attend various workshops and lectures on subjects they need to learn. These events also offer opportunities to meet with others facing the same or similar challenges and to learn from colleagues how to approach specific issues. In fact, ACMPE even requires its members to document 50 hours of continuing education over a three-year period to maintain certification.

▪ Credentialing and Leadership

Board certification of the medical practice executive acts as a demonstration of the executive's commitment to professionalism, and one of the common principles in all the definitions of professionalism is the necessity to participate in continuing education. By participating in continuing education, the executive makes a statement to the practice's partners, to colleagues, and to staff that the executive values the process of participating in continuing education and is thus of more value, with a higher skill set, than one who does not. As noted earlier, medical practice takes place in a highly credentialed environment, and by holding board certification, the executive demonstrates to the partners and staff a commitment to all of the values of professionalism, including the value of continuing education.

With physicians trained to deliver highly specialized patient care, partners are dependent upon the medical practice executive to arrange the business affairs of the practice to achieve the group's goals. Colleagues, both internal and external to the practice, must respect the executive's leadership skills for the practice to thrive. The old adage about the leader without followers is true: If people are unwilling to follow, leaders are unable to lead. Much of the willingness to follow is based on the trust placed in the executive's leadership. Followers, whether they be partners, colleagues, or staff, need to trust a leader's (the practice executive's) skills in order to fully participate in processes.

There are as many different leadership styles as there are leaders, but at some level, leaders have earned the trust of their followers through experience, respect, and special knowledge and skills. In a special 2004 *Business Week* report, "The Future of Work," those careers expected to survive and thrive in the future economy were those positions that required "flexibility, creativity and a commitment to life-long learning." [32] In contrast, positions with regularly recurring, routine work demands were expected to wither away. As cited by author Peter Coy in the *Business Week* report, in "The New Division of Labor: How Computers Are Creating the Next Job Market," Frank Levy of MIT and Richard J. Murnane of Harvard state that two kinds of jobs will remain in high demand. The first involves complex pattern recognition, such as spotting business opportunities or dealing with complex systems. The second category relies on complex communication skills, such as managing people, devising advertising campaigns, or selling big-ticket items. It is clear that a medical practice executive holds responsibilities similar to both of the types that are expected to thrive. In summary, the article's author, Peter Coy, states, "Are you flexible, creative and good with people? You should do fine in tomorrow's job market."[33] The leadership skills an executive develops and exhibits are often what differentiate the successful practice from those practices "just getting by."

TASK 2 # Balance Professional and Personal Pursuits

■ Work-Life Balance

Successful practice executives are usually motivated people, dedicated to their jobs and relentless in the pursuit of their business goals. However, this same personality trait carries with it a risk that the executive can become a workaholic because no medical practice ever seems to run out of opportunities for "just a little more time or management." Many executives even socialize with the partners of the practice and in that way turn social activities into opportunities for more work. To paraphrase a view that some might view as archaic, Jack Welch, the self-described workaholic ex-CEO of General Electric, says many companies give only lip service to a work-life balance and that "life-balance accommodations are only earned through performance."[34] Executives, then, have to develop the skill of separating their work lives from their personal lives.

In the past decade or so, a growing movement has emerged around the concept of "family-friendly" workplaces. Several magazines (*Fortune*, *Forbes*, and *Working Mother*, to name a few) give out annual awards for the best places to work, and the U.S. Department of Commerce even publishes guidelines on how employers can make their company environments more "family friendly." Although executives consider these initiatives in terms of the practices they run, executives should recognize the value of such actions for themselves, as well.

No practice benefits from having a tired, overworked, stressed-out leader. Certainly, executives work tired, work long hours, or experience high levels of stress at times, but successful executives recognize the value of rest and relaxation, and they know how to fit it into their lives. As part of being self-aware, executives know that if they do not manage the several components of their lives (work, family, and community) that imbalance can lead to health problems, poor judgments, and burnout. Despite living in a "24-7 world," the successful executive knows no individual can participate in the full 24-7 without negative consequences.

The process of fitting leisure into one's life is part of a larger process of executive self-assessment and career planning. The successful executive is aware of his or her own style of work and how that style relates to others within the practice. Many have completed the Myers-Briggs Type Indicator® personality inventory or some similar tool to determine how they relate to others and how they come to decisions. Knowing how one's own style relates to others, and how others' styles relate to oneself makes the executive a more successful and effective leader. Being able to vary how one relates to others based upon their personalities allows one to motivate change more effectively.

Self-awareness also allows the successful executive to utilize self-assessment skills to plan career changes. When building a continuing education plan around the *ACMPE Guide to the Body of Knowledge for Medical Practice Management*, the executive also is building a career plan for himself or herself. In today's work world, most successful individuals are expected to have a series of positions throughout their careers, as opposed to the one job for life, which was the hallmark of previous generations. Rather than building that job series as a "random walk," the successful practice executive carefully plans a succession of career-building steps. To be sure, the politics of medical practices today still create many unplanned or involuntary job changes, even for successful executives, but even in those cases an individual with a career plan will have a direction for the next step.

When contemplating those next steps, successful executives will utilize the networking skills addressed previously to investigate market opportunities, discuss possibilities with others, and plan steps based on perception and reality. Often, others' perceptions can help one better refine one's own self-assessment, which can then lead to better planning.

The last self-assessment task of the successful executive is the ability to manage time effectively. Most medical practice executives have a multitude of demands on their time. The ability to prioritize work and to focus efforts on the most high-yielding projects is critical to the executive's success. As previously discussed, the complexities of modern medical practice produce a plethora of opportunities to become a workaholic because there is always "just one more project" or "just one more thing" that requires attention. The successful executive knows that trying to solve all the issues or problems directed his or her way is like following the siren song of Odysseus. Only by truly prioritizing and selecting those projects with the highest potential yield will the executive's return on invested time and energy be maximized. The successful executive knows that some of the issues directed his or her way are not really the practice's problems and that other issues will resolve themselves without any action on the executive's part. By maximizing the executive's time on high-priority and high-yield projects, the executive's contribution to the practice is maximized.

TASK 3 **Promote Ethical Standards for Individual and Organizational Behavior and Decision Making**

■ Ethical Standards – The Heart of the Professional Responsibility Domain

As noted previously in the discussion of professionalism, one of the common threads in all definitions of professionals is adherence to an ethical standard and a definitive statement that individuals will act with integrity. Indeed, some definitions state that the members of a profession will act as ethical enforcement for the rest of the profession. Thus, attorneys have membership in their state bar associations as a prerequisite to licensure, and launch inquiries and investigations through the bar association when one member accuses another of acting unethically. Ethical standards require adherence to a higher standard of action than simple, expedient, and technically correct business actions. As discussed in the section on professional knowledge, ethical behavior requires adherence to duty and vigilance of action. Ethical behavior means actions are not only legal, but "right" from a variety of perspectives. In some cases, ethical behavior may actually increase the costs of doing business, not only from a vigilance perspective, but because actions are taken that would not be taken absent an ethical standard. In putting patients' interests above those of the practice, in some cases the practice may come out worse off economically. In treating staff fairly, as opposed to simply "what can be gotten away with," a practice sometimes will raise its costs. Investing in quality assurance programs because it is the right thing to do for patients can increase a practice's costs. Nevertheless, doing the right thing is a cost of doing business and is one that the professionally responsible medical practice executive recognizes.

Medical practices sometimes have competing goals, and if not held to high standards, those so-called "structural" conflicts can create opportunities for unethical behavior. Maximizing the partners' incomes can compete with goals of serving the community or treating the staff fairly, and it is up to the executive to uphold that higher standard and recognize and manage the potential conflicts of interest. The professional executive's sense of duty – to patients, to the partners, to the staff, and to the community – is sometimes the last line of defense guarding against unethical outcomes. Recently in Vermont, a hospital CEO was sentenced to two years in federal prison for lying to state regulators about the costs of a building expansion. By following his perceived *sole* duty to his employer to get state approval for the project at all costs, he violated ethical principles and even the law. Three others from that hospital's executive team also face criminal charges in that case.[35]

These types of cases illustrate that maintaining ethical standards is a matter of individual integrity and that only by being bound by a sense of professional responsibility and what is right or wrong will an executive truly rise to the level of a professional.

TASK 4 **Conduct Self-Assessments**

■ Self-Assessment Tools and Career Building

In addition to the ACMPE's online professional development assessment tools,[36] a variety of tools exist to help the medical practice executive identify gaps in skills sets and better understand his or her own strengths or weaknesses. As noted earlier, one particularly useful tool is the Myers-Briggs Type Indicator® personality profile.[37] Individuals use information drawn from this profile to assist with, among other things, career planning, improving negotiating skills, and enhancing daily interpersonal interactions. The book *Who Moved My Cheese?*, which was the number-one business best seller for months, focuses on how to manage change.[38] Other tools include the classic book *What Color Is Your Parachute? 2006*[39] along with such favored MGMA publications as *Take Charge of Your Health Care Career*[40] and *Take Charge of Your Employment Agreement*.[41]

Effectively using the information provided in job evaluations is critical for ongoing self-assessment. Listening to supervisors, subordinates, peers, friends, and family provides real-time feedback and contributes to the success of a professional. In a keynote address to the membership at an MGMA annual conference, Alan Stoll, FACMPE, called it "Me, Inc."[42] In his address, Stoll extolled the virtues of viewing oneself as a business product – a product that deserves as much attention as the medical practice (or organization) one manages.

The point is obvious; in the vernacular of today, the medical practice executive is a "product," one that should be under continuous quality improvement and one that is exposed to evaluative information 24-7. If this information is appropriately received and processed, smart decisions and continual self-improvement can occur. Moreover, the ability to recognize one's own strengths and weaknesses can lead to higher job satisfaction and improved work performance. As one expert says, "improving job performance relies more on organizing your life, getting enough rest and making sure you have good working conditions than on constant ... mind-breaking work."[43]

TASK 5 **Engage in Professional Networking**

■ Tapping into Networks

Given the complexity of the health care environment, the rapid pace of change, and the increasing specialization of the field, the medical practice executive's ability to tap into an informed network of colleagues and organizations is essential. Whether for physicians, allied health professionals, or medical practice leadership, professional organizations exist at all levels – local, regional, national, and even international. Professional organizations do not have to be limited, however, to the health care environment. Groups at the local level, such as Toastmasters, Jaycees, Rotary, and Lions Clubs, offer an excellent opportunity to network and participate in the business community at large. MGMA and ACMPE, along with their specialty societies and assemblies, offer opportunities at the state and national levels. Among other health care organizations are the Healthcare Financial Management Association (HFMA), the American College of Healthcare Executives (ACHE), and specialty society organizations such as the American College of Cardiology (ACC), and the American College of Obstetrics and Gynecology (ACOG).

Many an executive's reach has been measured by the power of his or her Rolodex or personal digital assistant (PDA) – objects that represent the ability to reach the right person, at the right place, at the right time. With PDAs so ubiquitous in today's business world, the term

"Rolodex" might seem archaic, conjuring up an image of a wheeled directory of names and phone numbers. But the idea of the power and capability to contact someone "in the know" through a quick phone call remains the same.

Certainly the power of the e-mail forum (e.g., Listserv®) has revolutionized business connectivity, linking individuals and groups of like interests electronically.[44] On an active electronic discussion list, industry news can be instantly distributed, questions can be asked and answered, and a repository of knowledge can be tapped.

In today's complex environment, then, when appropriately tapped, networks offer a powerful professional aid to the medical practice executive.

TASK 6 **Advance the
Profession by
Contributing to
the Body of
Knowledge**

■ Contributions to the Body of Knowledge

Perhaps the ultimate personal professional achievement
for the medical practice executive is the ability to trans-
late experience into contributions to a larger, collective
body of knowledge. Such contributions keep the profession current and relevant and advance the profession to a
higher level. Such contributions also force the contributor
to stay current, topical, and productive.

Many ways exist to contribute to the profession's
body of knowledge, and specifically to the medical practice management body of knowledge as defined by the
eight domains in the ACMPE *Guide*. Mentorship passes
along information at a personal level. Participating in
local "speaker's bureaus" expands the audience, as does
presenting information, research, or experiences at
regional or national conferences. Actively participating in
an e-mail forum is another tool for contributing – a tool
that might reach thousands internationally. Finally, making written contributions to newsletters, publications,
and books provides a way to "give back" to a profession
affected by so many.

Regardless of the method, contributing to the body of knowledge can be personally and professionally rewarding and helps to set and raise the standard for executives to follow.

TASK 7 # Develop Effective Interpersonal Skills

■ Group Dynamics and Interpersonal Skills

An executive who knows himself or herself will be a more effective leader and will recognize the importance of an interpersonal skill set that values and draws out individual and team contributions. Dispelling any doubt about the importance of honing interpersonal skills, the *Business Week* article mentioned earlier identified the ability to "manage people" as a skill set that would ensure an individual's future employment.[45]

The military has certainly understood the need to manage people as well as the value of teamwork. In his book, *Business Is Combat*, author James D. Murphy applies the lessons of a combat pilot to general business management.[46] Murphy points out that it is teams of people who get a fighter plane off the ground, and he lists techniques to improve teamwork, from clearly articulating a mission to punctuality (starting meetings on time) and exercising respect for colleagues (teammates).

Health care, by its very nature, is team-oriented; indeed, multidisciplinary teams deliver patient care. From the building maintenance staff to the operating room surgeon, scores, if not hundreds, of staff are involved in the safe and effective delivery of quality health care. The book *The Physician-Manager Alliance* states that "today ... the ethical provider is not a solitary physician but a complex health care organization operating under constraints that daily test their commitment to patients."[47] Team management, then, is a critical element in the medical practice executive's success. Effective leadership is the key to developing strong teams, and strong interpersonal skills serve as a foundation for this leadership.[48] Knowledge of team and interpersonal dynamics assists the executive in providing this leadership.

Vignette Redux

IN THE SCENARIO presented at the beginning of this volume, the medical practice executive is expected to comment on six physician or staff actions that will be presented to the group's executive committee for discussion. To review, the requests before the committee are to:

1. Temporarily lower compensation as a partner goes through a divorce settlement;

2. Defer compensation to mitigate another partner's taxes;

3. Increase self-referrals or charge higher fees to increase incentive compensation;

4. Lower charges for patients with no or limited ability to pay and conversely close another part of the practice to urban patients;

5. Approve an educational retreat and accept payment from a pharmaceutical company to finance part of it; and

6. Address a staff complaint about a partner's behavior.

This vignette highlights some of the breadth of knowledge and environmental sensitivity that is required of the professionally responsible medical practice executive.

Each action touches upon an area of professional responsibility, and how each one is addressed and the outcome of each can place the individual partners and certainly the practice at risk. Each of the issues identified could and should be reviewed at some length; the following points highlight some of the key considerations as well as some of the risks inherent in each request.

- *Lowering compensation in a divorce proceeding:* Partner One's request almost certainly raises an ethical question and might result in a civil legal action if the practice were to agree to allow the partner to manipulate her income with the obvious goal of hiding assets from her spouse. By almost all measures, the request is unethical and violates a "do the right thing" standard to which a medical practice executive subscribes. A clearly written compensation plan that is consistently administered will help shield the practice from such requests and guide the executive committee in its deliberation. Seeking advice from the practice's attorney would be another option before granting such a request.

- *Deferring compensation:* Partner Two's request to have his bonus check mailed in the new year as opposed to the current year is not necessarily illegal, unethical, or problematic. A clearly drafted compensation policy can help guide the practice on such requests. If Partner Two's goal is to move a taxable event into the next year, the medical practice executive should advise him to consult his accountant because the IRS might view the bonus as paid in 200X, even if the check is mailed in 200X+1, under its doctrine of "constructive receipt," which limits "the ability of cash basis taxpayers to arbitrarily shift income from one year to another in an effort to minimize total taxes."[49]

- *Boosting incentives through more self-referrals or higher fees and refusing to accept referrals from lower-paying patients from partners:* Partner Three's idea of increasing his bonus incentives through increased referrals to the hospital, ordering more medical labs or tests, or charging higher fees has problems on both ethical and legal levels. Ordering tests for personal gain that are potentially medically unnecessary is unethical and has social and economic implications for the patient, the practice, and the community at large. To do so would be a clear failure of one's duty to put the patients' interests first in all decisions about their care. Stark legislation and its proscriptions on self-referrals and suspicious physician-hospital relationships place the physician and the practice at risk. Charging higher fees at will causes billing compliance problems and opens the practice to negative repercussions from a governmental audit. At worst, a critical review of the proposed practices by the medical group's attorney is required. Refusing to accept referrals from partners based on patients' insurance status similarly puts the internal operations of the practice at risk. Essentially, this partner is putting his or her income desires in conflict with the group's decision to admit lower-paying patients to the practice by endangering the comity of practice operations and disregarding standing policies. A group practice ethos that discourages such behavior, supported by written principles and a clearly documented compensation plan, along with complementary policies and procedures – to include a uniform practice fee schedule – is the ideal.

- *Charging low income/no income patients lower fees:* Uniform fees and billing compliance are the issues here. Failure of either exposes the practice to sanctions in governmental audits. Establishing a uniform fee schedule, enforcing its use, and establishing uniform collection policies are defenses against potential abuses.

- *Drug company support of an educational retreat:* The American Medical Association (AMA) has adopted guidelines on accepting pharmaceutical support, gifts, and trips, and these should guide the practice in its decision making. There is no question that accepting the support creates at least an appearance of a conflict of interest between the physician's duty to patients and his or her later prescribing patterns based on such support. In addition, if the group is a nonprofit corporation, it needs to be aware that excessive compensation to its staff might make it vulnerable to "intermediate sanctions," a doctrine adopted by the IRS that addresses executives and staff who might be overpaid or can be influenced by inordinate payments, gifts, benefits, and trips offered to all employees of the practice.[50]

- *Staff complaint about the work environment:* The newest partner in the practice appears to have a style that is causing a staff complaint. Depending upon the result of an internal investigation of the staff member's circumstances, the practice might be accused of supporting a hostile work environment, opening it to an Equal Employment Opportunity Commission (EEOC) complaint and possible investigation, and potentially to a separate civil action should the staff member decide to engage an attorney on her own. To not take any action would be a clear failure of duty to employees to create a safe and secure working environment, as well as a potential failure of duty to the partners by putting the practice at legal risk. In either case, the practice is vulnerable to, at a minimum, losing a valuable employee and incurring the subsequent training and recruitment costs to replace her and, at worst, a damaging and costly lawsuit or judgment.

Conclusion

■ It Is Just Good Business

Whether it involves personal or professional growth, a strong sense of "fair play," avoiding legal and ethical circumstances, or simply "giving back" to the profession, the Professional Responsibility domain covers a wide range of skill sets that are interwoven with the other seven domains contained within the Technical/ Professional Knowledge and Skills General Competency for Medical Practice Management within the ACMPE *Guide*. Professional Responsibility involves developing and honing such skill sets as:

- Adhering to a set of values that demonstrate a professional code of ethics;

- Utilizing networks of colleagues and e-mail discussion lists to stay current and investigate new ideas, or simply to problem-solve;

- Continuing education to include self-study, board certification, and attendance at conferences or other group meetings in a variety of venues;

- Developing a knowledge of self through assessment, finding a work-life balance, and coping with information overload;

- Developing a set of tools that help manage people and changing systems;

- Contributing to the wider body of knowledge through mentoring, actively participating in networks, speaking, and publishing.

In short, Professional Responsibility is the overarching domain and is its own body of knowledge with its own set of skills that guide the medical practice executive through his or her professional life. As noted in the vignette, professional responsibility is also good risk management – management that preserves the integrity of the individual and the organization. Professional responsibility can inspire the medical executive and the practice to perform at a higher standard, benefiting the patient and the community at large. In fact, for the savvy medical practice executive, a keen sense of professional responsibility is just good business.

Exercises

THESE QUESTIONS have been retired from the ACMPE Essay Exam question bank. Because there are so many ways to handle various situations, there are no "right" answers, and thus no answer key. Use these questions to help you practice responses in different scenarios.

1. You are the new administrator for a small medical practice. You are new to the field of medical practice management and have worked in the accounting industry for several years. You would like to enhance your professional development in medical practice management.

   Develop and describe your career plan.

2. You are the chief executive officer of a large multispecialty group practice that has resulted from the recent merger and consolidation of three smaller practices. The group formed an executive committee that consists of a physician from each of the former practices. Conflict among the members of the executive committee has arisen over expense allocations.

    Discuss how you would work with the physician leaders to manage the conflict.

3. You are the administrator of a medical group. You are a member of a national health care professional association and were recently invited to serve on one of the organization's committees. You believe your service would help advance the profession and would like to serve. However, your supervisor is hesitant to approve your participation and is concerned that the time demands might interfere with your job duties.

    Describe how you would handle this situation.

4. You are the administrator of a three-physician single-specialty group, which is merging with another three-physician single-specialty group that has never employed an administrator. All six physicians have agreed that you should be the administrator for this new group, and you have accepted the position. Nevertheless, you feel the three new physicians are somewhat apprehensive about having a full-time administrator. In fact, a comment was made in the last meeting that they did not know what an "administrator" does.

    Describe how would you handle this situation.

5. You have been the administrator of a successful group practice for five years. However, managed care reimbursement is beginning to erode the income of physicians in your community. Many groups have attempted to reduce their administrative overhead. Several physicians in your group have expressed concern over what they perceive to be high administrative overhead. A physician has told you that several of the physicians feel that the administrative staff should be cut.

    Describe how would you handle this situation.

Notes

1. Mark Taylor, "Record Settlement. PharMerica Resolves Kickback Allegations," *Modern Healthcare* (April 4, 2005): 16.

2. Mark Taylor, "Medicaid Fraud Settled in N.Y.," *Modern Healthcare* (May 23, 2005): 12.

3. YAHOO, "Greenspan Urges Wharton Grads to Be Honest," www.yahoo.com/ap (retrieved May 16, 2005).

4. Ibid.

5. American College of Medical Practice Executives (ACMPE), *The ACMPE Guide to the Body of Knowledge for Medical Practice Management* (Englewood, Colo.: American College of Medical Practice Executives, 2003).

6. Milton H. Spencer, *Contemporary Economics* (New York: Worth Publishers, 1974), 33.

7. Malcolm Gladwell, *Blink: The Power of Thinking without Thinking* (New York: Little, Brown and Company, 2005), 8–10.

8. ACMPE, *The ACMPE Guide to the Body of Knowledge for Medical Practice Management*, 16.

9. Price Waterhouse Coopers, "The Sarbanes-Oxley Act," www.pwcglobal.com/Extweb (retrieved May 19, 2005).

10. "Compliance: Sarbanes-Oxley – Tech Listings," www.techlistings.net/xlist (retrieved May 19, 2005).

11. "Stark Law," en.wikipedia.org/wiki (retrieved May 20, 2005).

12. American Medical Directors Association (AMDA), "Guidance on Stark Law-Related Issues," www.amda.com/federalaffairs (retrieved May 20, 2005).

13. "The Aftermath," www.modernhealthcare.com (retrieved July 27, 2005).

14. "What is *Qui Tam?*" www.quitam.com/quitam1.html (retrieved May 19, 2005).

15. "*Respondeat Superior*" dictionary.law.com.definition2.asp (retrieved May 11, 2005).

16. Lawrence F. Wolper, ed., *Physician Practice Management: Essential Operational and Financial Knowledge* (Sudbury, Mass.: Jones and Bartlett Publishers, 2005), 472.

17. Laura Keidan Martin, "Excess Benefit Transactions," Education Session, Medical College of Wisconsin, 2003. Duplicated.

18. Ibid.

19. "Footnotes," The Statute Law Data Base by Roger Horne," www.number7.demon.co.uk/papers/SLD (retrieved May 23, 2005).

20. *Oxford English Dictionary*, http://dictionary.oed.com.

21. Jim Lakin, Nick Kupferle, Margie Jepson, & Andrea M. Rossiter, "MGMA and ACMPE Boards of Directors: Task Force on Professionalism." February 2005.

22. Florida Bar Association, "Center for Professionalism – Ideals and Goals of Professionalism," www.flabar.org/ (retrieved May 21, 2005). Emphasis added.

23. Accreditation Council of Graduate Medical Education (ACGME), "ACGME Outcome Project," www.acgme.org/outcome (retrieved May 11, 2005).

24. Australian Council of Professions, "Considerations about the Professionalism of Career and Transition Educators," www.cate.co.nz/CATEProf (retrieved May 11, 2005).

25. *Oxford English Dictionary.*

26. James D. Murphy, *Business Is Combat* (New York: HarperCollins Publishers, 2000), 36.

27. Thomas Sowell, *Applied Economics. Thinking Beyond Stage One* (Cambridge, Mass.: Perseus Books Group, 2004), 5.

28. Charles W. Hofer, Edwin A. Murray Jr., Ram Charan, & Robert A. Pitts, *Strategic Management* (St. Paul, Minn.: West Publishing Company, 1980), 12.

29. Barbara Bartlein, "Legendary Leaders Have Many Common Traits," *The Business Journal* (June 3, 2005): A18.

30. "Do the Right Thing," www.cinepad.com/reviews (retrieved May 19, 2005).

31. Cinda Becker, "CEOs Lose Jobs over Conflicts, Tests," *Modern Healthcare* (May 30, 2005): 12.

32. Peter Coy, "The Future of Work," *Business Week* (March 22, 2005): 50.

33. Ibid.

34. Jack Welch, with Suzy Welch, "From the Book *Winning*," *Newsweek* (April 4, 2005): 48.

35. Tony Fong, "Strong Message: Fletcher Allen Official Received Two-Year Sentence," *Modern Healthcare* (May 2, 2005): 17.

36. ACMPE offers a series of professional development assessments designed to evaluate an individual's knowledge within each of the eight performance domains defined in the *ACMPE Guide to the Body of Knowledge for Medical*

Practice Management. A description of each assessment is available in the Store section of the MGMA Website at www.mgma.com.

37. "The Myers-Briggs Type Indicator®," www.discoveryourpersonality.com/ MBTI (retrieved June 17, 2005).

38. Spencer Johnson and Kenneth H. Blanchard, *Who Moved My Cheese? An Amazing Way to Deal with Change in Your Work and in Your Life* (New York: Penguin Putnam Adult, 1998).

39. Richard Nelson Bolles, *What Color Is Your Parachute? 2006 (What Color Is Your Parachute?)* (Berkeley, Calif.: Ten Speed Press, 2005).

40. Hal Patterson, *Take Charge of Your Health Care Career: Successful Job-Search Strategies for the Health Care Professional* (Englewood, Colo.: Medical Group Management Association, 1998).

41. Hal Patterson, *Take Charge of Your Employment Agreement: A Win-Win Communication Tool for Medical Practice Executives,* (Englewood, Colo.: Medical Group Management Association, 2002).

42. David J. Peterson, "Taking Care of Me, Inc.," *AAP Grapevine* 12, no. 1 (Winter 1999): 11.

43. Blanca Torres, "It's the Little Things that Push Productivity Up, *Milwaukee Journal Sentinel* (May 15, 2005): 4D.

44. "Glossary of Selected Distance Learning Terms and Phrases," www. trainingfinder.org/DCD_lingo (retrieved June 17, 2005).

45. Coy, "The Future of Work," 50.

46. Murphy, *Business Is Combat*, 15.

47. Stephen M. Davidson, Marion McCollom, & Janelle Heineke, *The Physician-Manager Alliance* (San Francisco: Jossey-Bass, 1996), 72.

48. Patrick Lencioni, *The FIVE Dysfunctions of a TEAM.* (San Francisco: Jossey-Bass, 2002), 195.

49. Lawrence C. Phillips & William H. Hoffman Jr., eds., *West's Federal Taxation: Individual Income Taxes* (St. Paul, Minn.: West Publishing, 1980), 87.

50. Laura Keidan Martin, "Excess Benefit Transactions," Education Session. Medical College of Wisconsin, 2003. Duplicated.

51. "Intermediate Sanctions," en.wikipedia.org/wiki (retrieved June 17, 2005).

52. "What is *Qui Tam*?"

Glossary

Confidentiality – Protection of individually identifiable information from access by nonauthorized parties.

Body of Knowledge for Medical Practice Management (The) – Proper name for the collected information covering all aspects of the profession of medical practice management. The *ACMPE Guide to the Body of Knowledge for Medical Practice Management* identifies five key competencies: (1) Professionalism; (2) Leadership; (3) Communication Skills; (4) Organizational and Analytical Skills; and (5) Technical/Professional Knowledge and Skills. Within the Technical/Professional Knowledge and Skills competency are eight performance domains identified in the ACMPE Role Delineation Study as being critical to a successful medical practice executive: (1) Financial Management; (2) Human Resource Management; (3) Planning and Marketing; (4) Information Management; (5) Risk Management; (6) Governance and Organizational Dynamics; (7) Business and Clinical Operations; and (8) Professional Responsibility.

Constructive receipt – An Internal Revenue Service doctrine that identifies when the recipient of income actually needs to report the income.

E-mail forum – An online discussion group whose participants exchange messages of common interest. (Also called a *newsgroup, bulletin board, or online conference*).

HIPAA (Health Insurance Portability and Accountability Act of 1996) – Sweeping health care legislation adopted in 1996 geared toward protecting health care information, setting standards for business transactions between health care entities, and establishing rules for insurance portability.

Intermediate Sanctions – An Internal Revenue Service term that is "applied to nonprofit organizations who engage in transactions that inure to the benefit of a *disqualified person* within the organization … allowing the IRS to penalize the organization and the disqualified person receiving the benefit."[51]

Invisible hand – Economist Adam Smith's idea presented in *The Wealth of Nations* that each individual will achieve the "best good for society" if allowed to pursue his or her self-interest without government interference.

Myers-Briggs Type Indicator® – A psychological test designed to assist a person in identifying his or her personality preferences.

Qui tam – Latin term for a provision in the federal Civil False Claims Act "that allows private citizens to file a lawsuit in the name of the U.S. government charging fraud."[52]

Respondeat superior – Latin for "let the master answer," and a doctrine of law that might hold the employer liable for his or her employees' actions in the course of employment.

Safe harbors – A legal provision to reduce or eliminate liability; safe harbors are identified in the Federal Anti-Kickback statute.

Sarbanes-Oxley Act – Signed into law in 2002, this legislation holds publicly traded companies more accountable to investors, auditors, and the public at large.

Stark Law – Law named for Congressman Pete Stark (D-CA) that governs physician self-referral for Medicare and Medicaid patients.

501(c) 3 – Internal Revenue Service designation (from the section of the code) that describes a nonprofit organization.

About the Authors

David Peterson, MBA, FACMPE, is a credentialed administrator for the Department of Psychiatry & Behavioral Medicine at the Medical College of Wisconsin. He is responsible for a $25 million multidisciplinary department comprising more than 200 faculty, staff, and residents active in patient care, NIH-funded research, and teaching programs. Mr. Peterson is active in ACMPE, having served as an examiner, as a team leader, and as chair of the ACMPE Professional Papers Committee. His publications on business and health care include papers on topics as diverse as desktop computing and human resource management, a recent article on leadership skills in the *ACMPE Executive View™*, and a chapter on budgeting for a book published by the American Psychiatric Press. He also writes a regular column for his specialty group newsletter.

After his honorable discharge from the U.S. Army, Mr. Peterson earned a bachelor of science degree in Business Administration and a master of business administration degree, both from the University of South Dakota. He is a member of two business and economic honor societies, Beta Gamma Sigma and Omicron Delta Epsilon. Prior to his work in health care, Mr. Peterson worked as an analyst for a Fortune 100 company.

Ken Mace, MA, CMPE, is the administrator of the Department of Family and Community Medicine at the Medical College of Wisconsin. His experience includes more than 20 years in health care planning and management, medical education, and ambulatory services administration. Prior to joining the Medical College, Mr. Mace was associate administrator for ambulatory services at West Suburban Hospital in Oak Park, Illinois. He worked in a variety of roles at Broadlawns Medical Center in Des Moines, Iowa, a large public hospital and ambulatory services center, eventually becoming associate director. Preceding this experience, he served as an administrator in the University of Iowa College of Medicine.

Mr. Mace has authored or co-authored several articles related to medical education and ambulatory care administration, and he is a frequent speaker at national conferences, presenting seminars and workshops on these topics. He earned a bachelor's degree in Communications and Political Science from the University of Iowa and spent several years in health and hospital planning positions before returning to the University of Iowa to receive a master's degree in Hospital and Health Administration.

Index

Accreditation Council for Graduate Medical Education (ACGME), 13, 56
American College of Healthcare Executives (ACHE), 37
American College of Medical Practice Executives (ACMPE)
  essay exam, 49
  Guide, 14-16, 20, 30, 39, 47, 59
  role delineation study, 59
American Medical Association (AMA), 45
Australian Council of Professions, 13

Balance professional and personal pursuits, 21, 29-31
Business Week, 26, 28, 41

Career building, 30, 35
Certified Medical Practice Executive (CMPE), ix, 61
Change management, 26
Changing information requirements, 25
Civil False Claims Act, 60
Colleagues, 17-18, 27, 37, 41, 47
Communication skills, 5, 28, 59
Compliance, 45, 55
Confidentiality, 13, 18, 59
Conflict, 19, 34, 45, 50
Constructive receipt, 44, 59
Continuing education, 8, 14, 16, 26-27, 30, 47
Credentialing, 27
Current professional responsibility issues, 7-9

Decision making, 5, 20, 22, 33, 45

E-mail, 38-39, 47, 59
Education needs, 21
Equal Employment Opportunity Commission (EEOC), 46
Ethical standards, promoting, 22, 23
Ethics, 1, 13-14, 18-19, 22, 33, 47

Failure, 8, 11, 45, 46
Federal
  Anti-Kickback Statute, 8, 60
  Reserve Board, xi
Financial management, xii, 26, 37, 59
Followers, 27-28
Forbes, 29
Fortune, 29

Governance, 5, 7, 59
Greenspan, Alan, xi, xii
Group dynamics, 41
Groups, 26, 37-38, 53

Health care professional, 51, 57, 59
Health Insurance Portability and Accountability Act (HIPAA), 7, 15, 59
Healthcare Financial Management Association (HFMA), 26, 37

Incentives, 3, 19, 44
Information
  management, 16, 59
  networking,17
  overload management, 16
  requirements, 25
Information technology (IT), 4, 9, 11-17, 19-22, 25-26, 28-30, 34-35, 41, 43, 45-47, 57